# NATHAN S. YORK

# Understanding Kidney Stones

*Your Top Questions With Simple Answers!*

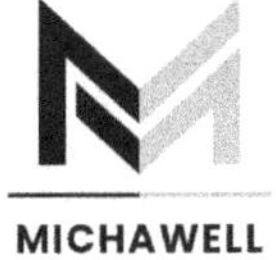

**MICHAWELL**

# Contents

# 1

# Introduction

Understanding kidney stones is crucial as it empowers you to prevent and manage this common condition, which can be very painful and distressing. This guide is designed to provide you with the knowledge you need to take control of your kidney health.

Learning about kidney stones can help you take steps to prevent them and seek proper treatment if you develop them. This guide will cover what kidney stones are, how they form, the symptoms they cause, how they are diagnosed and treated, and how to prevent them. You'll also learn about the different types of kidney stones, the role of the kidneys in your body, and the impact of diet and hydration on kidney stone formation.

By understanding kidney stones, you can make informed decisions about your health and take steps to reduce your risk. Whether you are a patient, a medical professional, or want to learn more about kidney health, this guide will provide valuable information. Please note, however, that this book is designed to provide basic information about kidney stones. For more detailed information, please consult a healthcare professional.

# 2

# Can You Tell Me About the Kidneys?

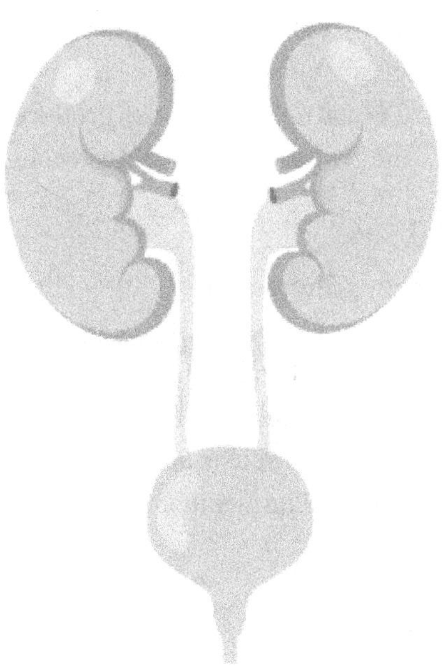

*Kidneys with ureters and bladder*

### What are the kidneys?

Before we delve into kidney stones, it's essential to understand the kidneys and their role in the urinary tract. The kidneys, two bean-shaped organs located in your lower back, perform several vital functions that are crucial for your overall health:

- **Filter Waste:** The kidneys filter waste products and excess fluids from your blood, which are then excreted as urine.
- **Balance Fluids:** They help balance the levels of fluids and electrolytes in your body.
- **Regulate Blood Pressure:** The kidneys produce hormones that help regulate blood pressure.
- **Produce Red Blood Cells:** They also produce a hormone that stimulates the production of red blood cells.

### How do the kidneys filter waste?

The kidneys filter waste through tiny structures called nephrons. Each kidney has about a million nephrons. Blood flows into the nephrons, where waste products and excess fluids are removed and turned into urine. The clean blood is then returned to the body.

### Where does the urine go?

The urine is drained from each kidney down a tube called a ureter. Each kidney and ureter drain into the bladder, where the urine is collected. The urine is then transported out of the body through the urethra.

# 3

# What Should You Know About Kidney Stones?

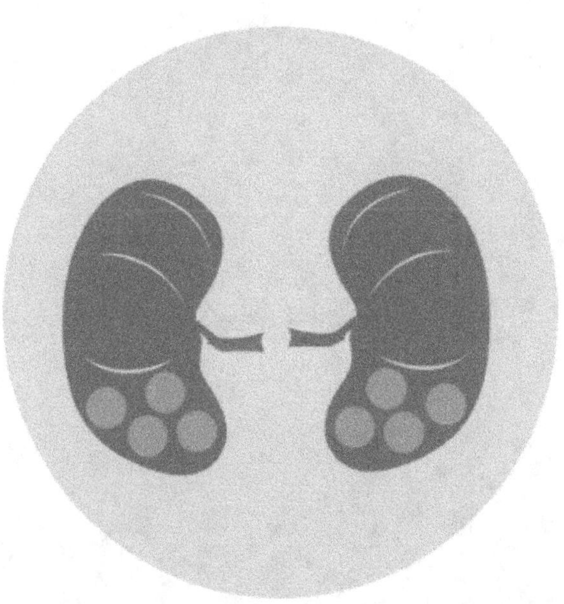

*Stones in the kidneys*

**What are kidney stones?**

Kidney stones, hard lumps made of minerals and salts, can cause significant discomfort and health issues. They can be as small as a grain of sand to as large as a golf ball, underscoring the urgency of prevention and treatment.

**Where do kidney stones come from?**

Kidney stones form inside the kidneys when too many minerals are in the urine. The minerals stick together to form stones.

**How do kidney stones form?**

Kidney stones form when certain substances in your urine, like calcium, oxalate, and uric acid, become too concentrated. When these substances stick together, they form crystals. Over time, these crystals can grow into a stone.

**Why do these substances stick together?**

Normally, your urine contains chemicals that prevent these substances from sticking together. But if you don't drink enough water or eat foods that are high in these substances, the chemicals can't do their job, and stones can form.

# 4

# What Are the Symptoms of Kidney Stones?

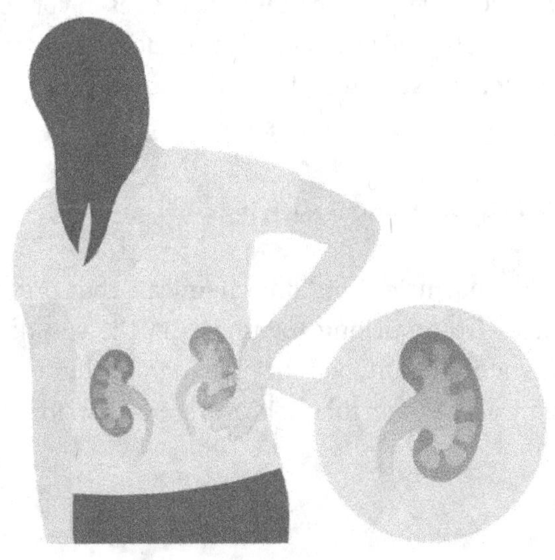

**What do you feel when you have a kidney stone?**

The most common symptom of kidney stones is severe pain, typically in your back, side, or lower belly. You might also experience pain during urination, blood in your urine, nausea, vomiting, and frequent urination. Recognizing these symptoms can help you seek timely treatment.

**Can kidney stones cause other problems?**

Kidney stones can cause infections in the kidneys or urinary tract. They can also block the flow of urine, which can damage the kidneys.

# 5

# How Are Kidney Stones Diagnosed?

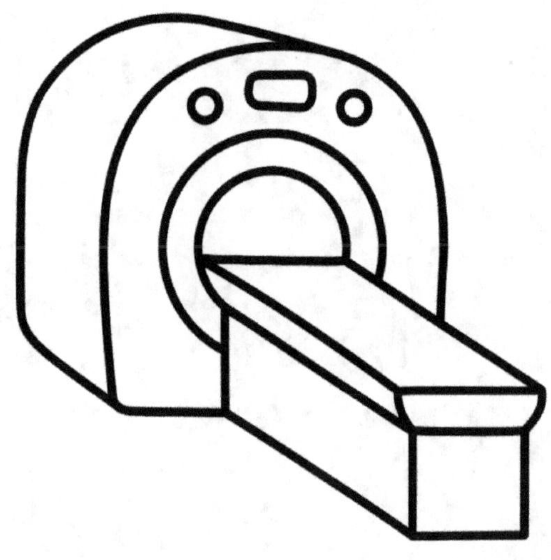

*A CT scan*

**How do doctors know if you have kidney stones?**

Doctors use several tests to determine whether you have kidney stones. These tests include urine tests, blood tests, X-rays, and CT scans. They help doctors see the stones and check for other problems.

**What is a CT scan?**

A CT scan is a special X-ray that takes detailed pictures of your kidneys and urinary tract.  It helps doctors see the size and location of the stones.

**What is an abdominal x-ray?**

An abdominal X-ray is a type of X-ray that takes pictures of the organs and structures in your abdomen, including the kidneys, ureters, and bladder. It can help doctors see some kidney stones, but not all rocks appear on X-rays.

**What is a kidney ultrasound?**

A kidney ultrasound is a test that uses sound waves to create pictures of your kidneys and urinary tract. It is a non-invasive and painless way to see kidney stones and check for other kidney and bladder problems.

# 6

# Are Stones Only Found in the Kidneys Themselves?

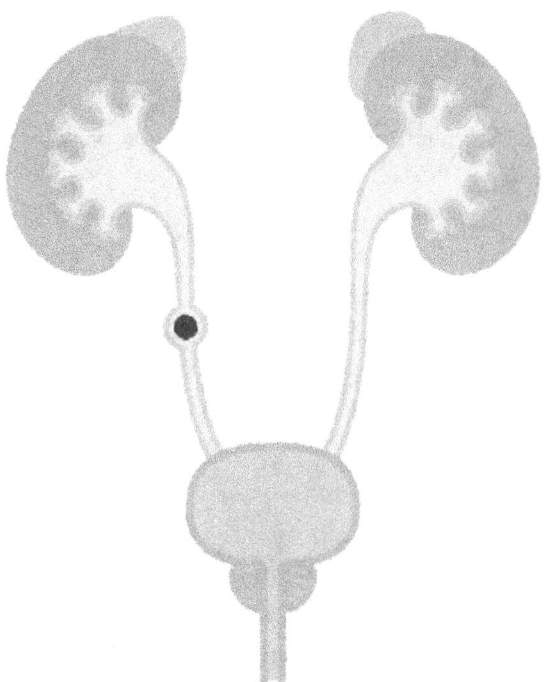

*A stone in the ureter causing obstruction of urine*

## Where can kidney stones be found in the urinary tract?

Kidney stones can occur anywhere in the urinary tract, including the kidneys, ureters, bladder, and urethra.

- **Kidneys:** Stones often form in the kidneys, where they can cause pain and blockages.

- **Ureters:** These tubes carry urine from the kidneys to the bladder. Stones can get stuck in the ureters, causing severe pain and blocking urine flow.
- **Bladder:** Stones can move from the kidneys or ureters into the bladder. They can cause pain and problems with urination.
- **Urethra:** The urethra is the tube that carries urine out of the body. Stones that pass into the urethra can cause intense pain and difficulty urinating.

**What happens if a stone gets stuck in the ureter?**

If a stone gets stuck in the ureter, it can block urine flow from the kidney to the bladder. This can cause severe kidney pain and swelling and potentially lead to infection or kidney damage.

# 7

## Who Takes Care of Kidney Stones?

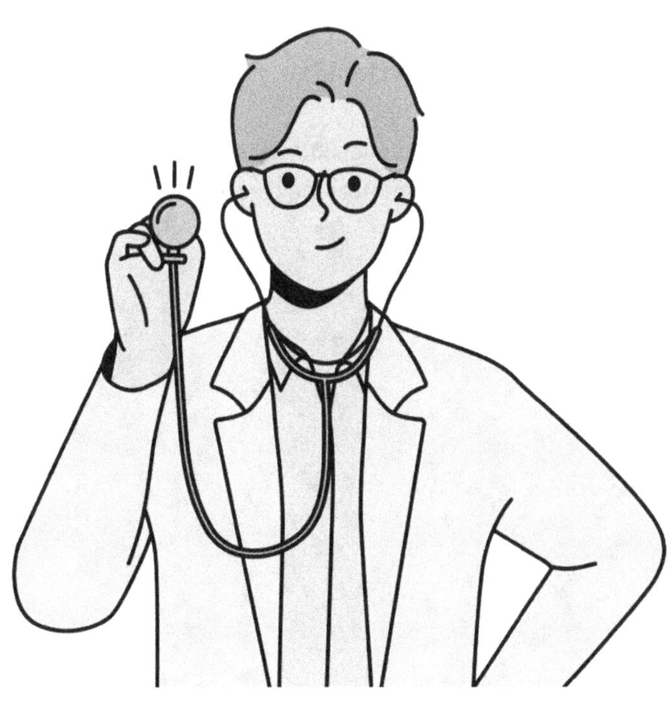

**Who should you see for kidney stones?**

If you think you have kidney stones, you should see a urologist. A urologist is a doctor who specializes in the urinary tract and male reproductive system. You may also see a nephrologist, a doctor who specializes in kidney care.

**What can a urologist do for kidney stones?**

A urologist can diagnose and treat kidney stones. They can perform procedures like lithotripsy or ureteroscopy to remove stones. They can also help you develop a plan to prevent future stones.

**What can a nephrologist do for kidney stones?**

A nephrologist can help manage kidney stones and any related kidney problems. They can provide treatments and advice to keep your kidneys healthy and prevent future stones.

# 8

# Is There a Treatment for Kidney Stones?

**How are kidney stones treated?**

Treatment depends on the size and type of stone. Small stones can often be passed by drinking lots of water and taking pain medicine. Larger stones may need to be broken up or removed by a doctor.

**What is an alpha-blocker?**

An alpha-blocker medication, such as tamsulosin (Flomax), helps relax specific muscles and keep small blood vessels open. Kidney stones, particularly smaller stones, can sometimes pass through the urinary tract independently. Alpha-blockers help this process by relaxing the muscles in the ureter, which allows the stones to pass more efficiently and with less pain.

# 9

# What Are Some Surgical Options?

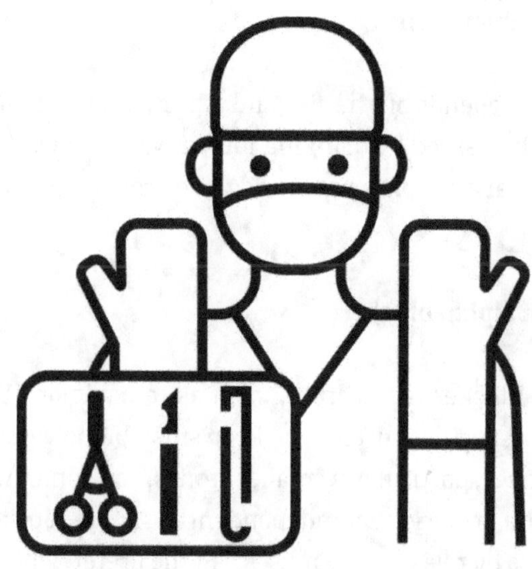

## What is a lithotripsy?

Lithotripsy is a medical procedure that breaks down kidney stones and in the urinary tract so they can be passed more easily. There are several types of lithotripsy, each using different methods to fragment the stones:

### 1. Extracorporeal Shock Wave Lithotripsy (ESWL)

ESWL uses shock waves generated outside the body to break kidney stones into smaller pieces that can be passed in the urine.

*Advantages:*

- Non-invasive.
- It can be performed on an outpatient basis.

*Disadvantages:*

- It is effective not only for some types of stones but also for large stones.
- It may require multiple sessions.
- Potential for discomfort or pain.

### 2. Ureteroscopy with Laser Lithotripsy

A ureteroscope (a thin tube with a camera) is inserted into the urethra, the bladder, and the ureter or kidney. A laser is then used to break up the stone.

*Advantages:*

- It can treat stones in the kidney, ureter, and bladder.
- High success rate for stone clearance.

*Disadvantages:*

- Invasive procedure.
- Requires anesthesia.
- Risk of ureteral injury or infection.

## 3. Percutaneous Nephrolithotomy (PCNL)

This surgical procedure involves making a small incision in the back to insert a nephroscope directly into the kidney. Ultrasonic or pneumatic energy is then used to break up the stone.

*Advantages:*

- Effective for large or complex stones.
- High success rate for stone removal.

*Disadvantages:*

- Invasive procedure with a longer recovery time.
- Higher risk of complications compared to other methods.
- Requires hospitalization.

## 4. Electrohydraulic Lithotripsy (EHL)

Uses electrical energy to create shock waves that break up stones. It is typically used in combination with endoscopic procedures like ureteroscopy.

*Advantages:*

- Effective for a variety of stone types.
- It can be used in the kidney, ureter, and bladder.

*Disadvantages:*

- Invasive.
- Requires anesthesia.
- Potential for tissue damage.

# What Are Other Procedures You May Hear About?

**What is a ureteral stent?**

A ureteral stent is a tube inserted into the ureter. Its primary purpose is to ensure the flow of urine from the kidney to the bladder, especially when the ureter is obstructed or at risk of becoming blocked.

**Purpose and Uses**

- Relieving Obstruction: Ureteral stents are often used to relieve obstructions caused by kidney stones. You may also hear them referenced when someone has a tumor, strictures (narrowing of the ureter), or other type of compression.
- Post-Surgical Support: They are commonly placed after surgeries involving the urinary tract to ensure that the ureter remains open and urine can flow freely while the

area heals.

- Facilitating Stone Passage: Stents can help reduce the passage of kidney stones by keeping the ureter open and allowing smaller fragments to pass more quickly.
- Preventing Urine Backflow: In certain medical conditions, stents can prevent urine from flowing back into the kidney, which could cause damage.

## What is a percutaneous nephrostomy?

A percutaneous nephrostomy involves inserting a catheter (a thin tube) directly into the kidney through the skin to drain urine. This may be performed by a doctor called an interventional radiologist. It is typically done when there is a blockage in the urinary tract from a stone that needs to be immediately relieved (when someone has a severe infection from a stone). It typically is a temporary procedure to allow the urinary system to heal with a plan for eventual further surgery.

## What procedure is right for me?

Each type of procedure has its own indications, advantages, and disadvantages. The choice of method depends on a number of factors including your overall health and preferences. You should discuss this with your urologist.

# 11

# What Happens After You Have a Stone?

**What happens after a kidney stone is removed?**

After a kidney stone is removed, your doctor will instruct you to prevent future stones. This may include drinking more water, changing your diet, and taking medications.

**Can you get kidney stones again?**

Yes, people who have had kidney stones are at higher risk of getting them again. Following your doctor's advice is essential to prevent future stones.

# 12

# What Are the Different Types of Kidney Stones?

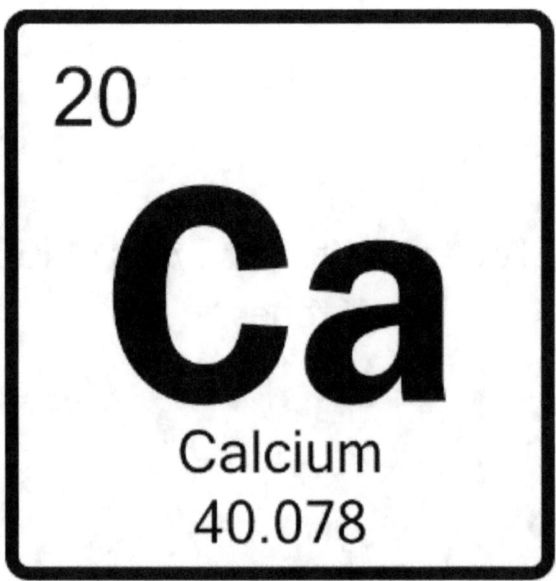


**Are there different types of kidney stones?**

Yes, there are four main types of kidney stones: calcium stones, uric acid stones, struvite stones, and cystine stones.

**What are calcium stones?**

Calcium stones are the most common type of kidney stone. They are made of calcium oxalate or calcium phosphate. These stones form when too much calcium or oxalate is in your urine.

### *Calcium Oxalate Stones*

Calcium oxalate stones are the most common type of kidney stone. They form when there is too much calcium and oxalate in the urine. Oxalate is found in many foods, such as spinach, nuts, and chocolate.

### *Calcium Phosphate Stones*

Calcium phosphate stones form when there is too much calcium and phosphate in the urine. These stones are less common than calcium oxalate stones.

## What are uric acid stones?

Uric acid stones form when too much uric acid is in your urine. This can happen if you eat a lot of meat, fish, or shellfish. Uric acid is a waste product usually dissolved in urine, but it can form stones if you have too much. Uric acid stones do not show up on regular X-rays.

## What are struvite stones?

Struvite stones form when you have a urinary tract infection. These stones are made of magnesium, ammonium, and phosphate. They can grow huge and cause problems with your kidneys.

## What are cystine stones?

Cystine stones are rare. They form in people who have a genetic disorder called cystinuria, which causes too much cystine in the urine.  Cystine is an amino acid that can form stones when it builds up in the urine.

# 13

# Why May You Have Kidney Stones?

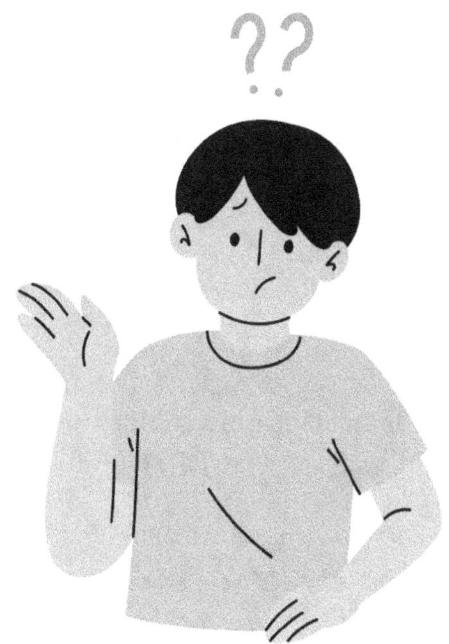

**What causes kidney stones?**

Kidney stones can be caused by not drinking enough water, eating a diet high in certain substances, being overweight, having certain medical conditions, and taking certain medications.

**What conditions are associated with kidney stones?**

Several conditions are associated with kidney stones, including dehydration, urinary tract infections, gout, and certain metabolic disorders. Conditions that affect how your body processes certain substances can also increase your risk of kidney stones.

**Can genetic factors increase the risk of kidney stones?**

Yes, genetic factors can increase the risk of kidney stones. If you have a family history of kidney stones, you may be more likely to develop them.

**What is cystinuria?**

Cystinuria is a genetic disorder that causes too much cystine in the urine. Cystine is an amino acid that can form stones when it builds up. People with cystinuria are at higher risk of developing cystine stones.

**Can eating certain foods cause kidney stones?**

Eating foods high in oxalate, such as spinach, nuts, and chocolate, can increase your risk of developing kidney stones. Eating too much salt or sugar can also contribute to stone formation.

**Can protein sources contribute to kidney stones?**

Eating a lot of animal protein, including red meat, poultry, and seafood, can increase your risk of developing kidney stones. Animal protein can increase the amount of uric acid in your urine which leads to uric acid stones.

**What is gout, and how is it related to kidney stones?**

Gout is a form of arthritis caused by high levels of uric acid in the blood. Uric acid can form crystals in the joints, leading to pain and inflammation. High levels of uric acid can also lead to the formation of uric acid kidney stones.

**What are metabolic disorders?**

Metabolic disorders affect how your body processes certain substances, such as calcium, oxalate, and uric acid. Examples include hyperparathyroidism and renal tubular acidosis. These disorders can increase your risk of developing kidney stones.

**Can malabsorptive conditions increase the risk of kidney stones?**

Yes, conditions that affect how your body absorbs nutrients, like Crohn's disease or gastric bypass surgery, can increase the risk of kidney stones. These conditions can cause changes in how your body processes calcium and oxalate, leading to stone formation.

# 14

# How Can You Prevent Kidney Stones?

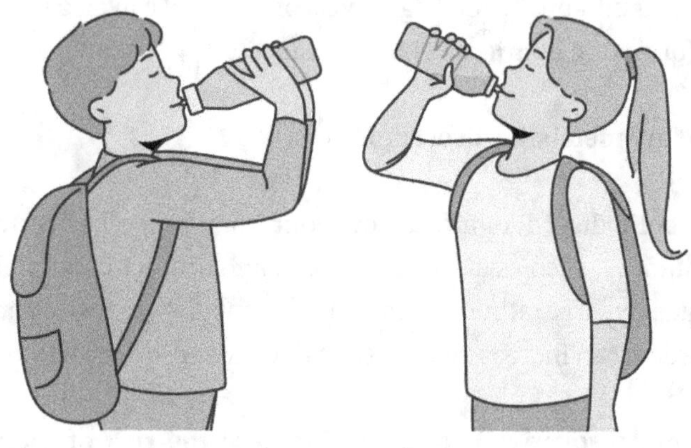

**How Do You Stop Future Kidney Stones from Forming?**

You can prevent kidney stones by drinking plenty of water and eating a balanced diet. Your doctor may also recommend medications to help prevent stones. We will discuss this with the following questions and answers.

**Why is drinking water essential for preventing kidney stones?**

Drinking water helps flush out the substances in your urine that can form stones. It also helps dilute your urine, making it harder for stones to form.

**How much water should I be drinking?**

With kidney stones, it is recommended to drink at least 2 liters of fluid per day, if not more. This is around eight 8-ounce glasses of water or about half a gallon per day.

**How do you know if you're drinking enough water?**

You know you drink enough water if your urine is light yellow or clear. If it is dark yellow, you are not drinking enough water.

# 15

# Should You Follow a Certain Diet?

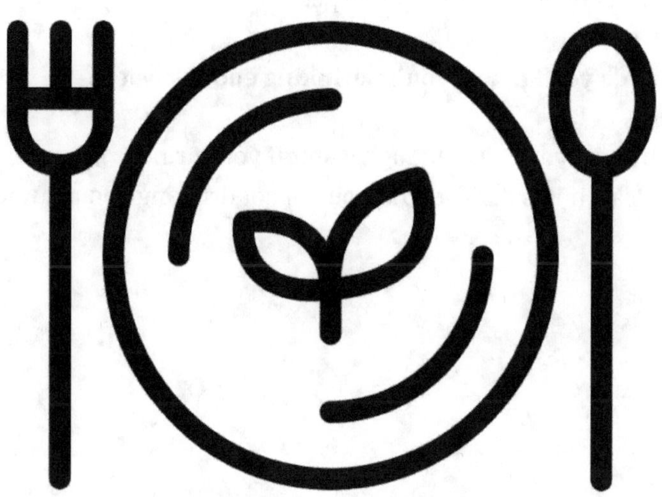

**What foods should you eat to prevent kidney stones?**

To prevent kidney stones, eat a diet high in fruits and vegetables, whole grains, and lean proteins. Avoid foods high in oxalate. Limit your intake of salt, sugar, and animal proteins (especially with uric acid stones).

**What are examples of foods that are high in oxalate?**

Foods high in oxalate can increase your risk of developing kidney stones. Here are some examples:

1. Vegetables: Spinach, rhubarb, beets, beet greens, Swiss chard, and sweet potatoes.
2. Fruits: Star fruit and raspberries.
3. Nuts and Seeds: Almonds, cashews, peanuts, and sesame seeds.
4. Grains: Wheat bran and buckwheat.
5. Legumes: Soybeans and tofu.
6. Other Foods: Dark chocolate, cocoa powder, and black tea.

**Should you avoid all high-oxalate foods?**

You don't need to avoid all high oxalate foods but eating them in moderation is essential if you are at risk for kidney stones.

**What about calcium?**

Most adults' recommended daily calcium intake is about 1,000 milligrams, but this can vary based on age and health conditions. It's important to get your calcium from dietary sources. Restricting calcium can lead to increased oxalate absorption, which increases the risk of calcium oxalate stones. However, too much calcium increases the calcium in the urine and leads to an increased risk of calcium stones in general.

**My doctor wanted me to take calcium with meals, so I thought I should take only a little calcium.**

Calcium binds to oxalate in the stomach and intestines before it reaches the kidneys. This helps reduce the amount of oxalate in urine. However, if your doctor recommends this if the benefits of binding oxalate increase the risk of more calcium in the urine, it should only be done.

# 16

# What Other Dietary Measures Should You Follow?

**How does a low-sodium diet help prevent kidney stones?**

A low-sodium diet helps prevent kidney stones by reducing the amount of calcium in your urine. High sodium intake can cause your kidneys to excrete more calcium, which can combine with oxalate or phosphate to form stones. Reducing sodium in your diet can help lower the risk of stone formation.

**What are some tips for following a low-sodium diet?**

*To follow a low-sodium diet, try these tips:*

- Read Labels: Look for foods labeled as low sodium or no salt added.
- Cook at Home: Prepare meals to control the salt you use.
- Avoid Processed Foods: Processed and packaged foods often

contain high sodium levels.

- Use Herbs and Spices: Flavor your food with herbs and spices instead of salt.
- Limit Fast Food: Fast and restaurant meals are often high in sodium.

**How do protein sources affect kidney stones?**

Eating a lot of animal protein, such as red meat, poultry, and seafood, can increase your risk of developing kidney stones. Animal protein can increase the amount of uric acid in your urine, which can lead to the formation of uric acid stones. It can also increase calcium excretion, raising the risk of calcium stones.

**What are uric acid sources?**

Uric acid is a waste product formed from the breakdown of purines found in many foods, especially animal proteins.

**Foods high in purines include:**

- Red Meat: Beef, pork, and lamb.
- Seafood: Shellfish, sardines, anchovies, and mackerel.
- Organ Meats: Liver, kidneys, and sweetbreads.
- Certain Vegetables: Asparagus, mushrooms, and spinach (though these are less likely to cause problems than animal sources).

**How can you limit uric acid sources?**

***To limit uric acid sources and reduce the risk of uric acid stones:***

- Reduce Animal Protein Intake: Eat smaller meat, poultry, and seafood portions.
- Choose Plant-Based Proteins: Opt for beans, lentils, tofu, and other plant-based proteins.
- Limit High-Purine Foods: Reduce or avoid foods high in purines, especially organ meats and certain seafood.
- Increase Dairy Intake: Dairy products can help lower uric acid levels.
- Drink Plenty of Water: Staying hydrated helps dilute the uric acid in your urine.

**Are There Any Drinks That Can Help Prevent Kidney Stones?**

Drinking lemonade made with natural lemon or lime juice can help prevent kidney stones. The citric acid in these drinks can help prevent stones from forming. However, ensure this is lemonade or limeade without high fructose corn syrup.

# 17

# Are There Medications to Take to Prevent Kidney Stones?

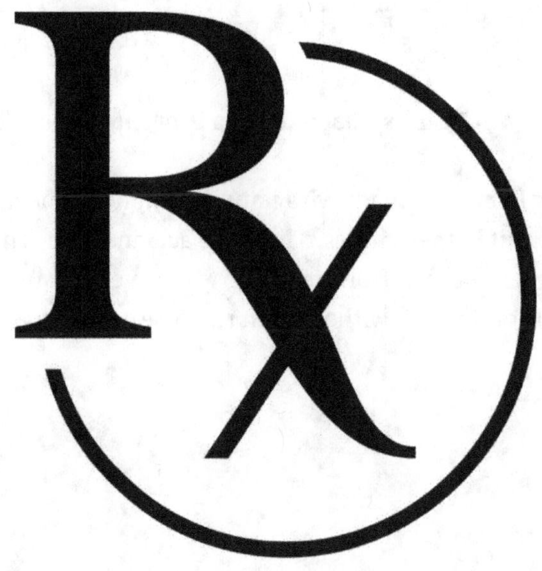

## What Can You Take to Prevent Stone Formation?

### *Thiazide Diuretics:*

- Examples: Hydrochlorothiazide, Chlorthalidone
- Purpose: To decrease calcium levels in the urine and prevent calcium stones.
- Considerations: May require potassium supplementation.

### *Potassium Citrate:*

- Purpose: To alkalize the urine, making it less acidic and preventing the formation of uric acid and cystine stones.
- Effectiveness: Useful in patients with a history of uric acid or cystine stones.

### *Allopurinol:*

- Purpose: To reduce uric acid levels and prevent uric acid stones.
- Considerations: Often used in conjunction with dietary modifications.

### *Antibiotics:*

- Examples: Long-term antibiotics may be necessary for struvite stones
- Purpose: To treat and prevent urinary tract infections

leading to stone formation.

There are other medications used in certain situations that are beyond the scope of this book.

# 18

# Are There Any Complications from Kidney Stones?

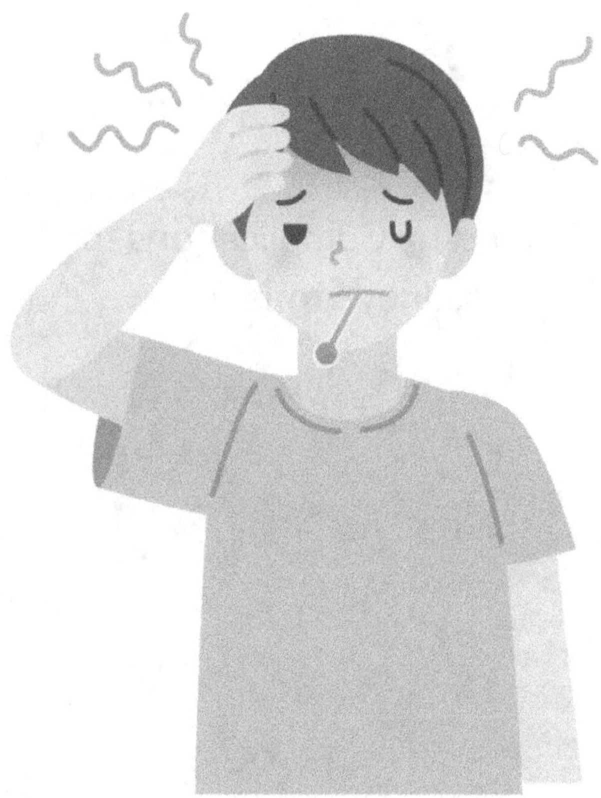

## Can kidney stones cause complications?

Kidney stones can cause complications if they block urine flow or cause an infection. These complications can damage your kidneys and may require emergency treatment.

## What are some signs of complications?

Signs of complications include severe pain, fever, chills, and difficulty urinating.  If you have any of these symptoms, you should immediately see a doctor.

# 19

# Can Everyone Get Kidney Stones?

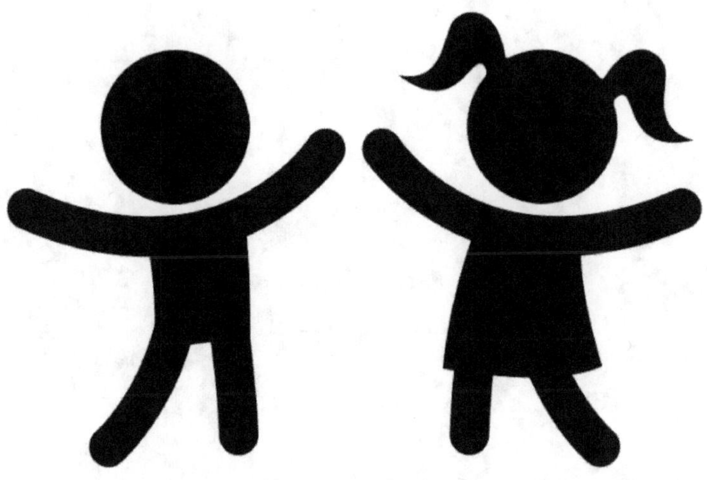

**Can kids get kidney stones?**

Yes, kids can get kidney stones, although it is less common than in adults. Kids without drinking enough water or having certain medical conditions are at higher risk.

**What should kids do to prevent kidney stones?**

Kids should drink plenty of water, eat a balanced diet, and avoid foods high in oxalate. They should also stay active and maintain a healthy weight.

20

# What Should You Do If You Think You Have a Kidney Stone?

**Should I Ignore This?**

No! If you think you have a kidney stone, you should see a doctor right away. They can perform tests to determine whether you have a stone and recommend the best treatment.

**Can you treat kidney stones at home?**

Small stones can sometimes be treated at home by drinking plenty of water and taking pain medicine. But you should always see a doctor to make sure you don't have a larger stone or other problems. Patients with liver disease, chronic kidney disease, and other medical conditions, such as stomach problems, should check with their medical provider before taking over-the-counter pain medications.

# 21

# Conclusion

Understanding kidney stones is the first step in preventing and managing this painful condition. By learning about how kidney stones form, their symptoms, and the different types of rocks, you can take proactive measures to reduce your risk. This guide has provided essential information on diagnosis, treatment options, and preventative strategies, all aimed at helping you maintain better kidney health.

Kidney stones can affect anyone, but staying informed and making healthy lifestyle choices can significantly lower your chances of developing them. Drinking plenty of water, following a balanced diet, and being mindful of your intake of high-oxalate and high-purine foods are crucial. If you ever experience symptoms of kidney stones, seeking medical attention promptly to receive the appropriate diagnosis and treatment is essential.

Remember, your kidneys are vital to your overall health, filtering waste and balancing fluids. Taking care of your kidneys means taking care of your entire body. By implementing the knowledge and tips in this guide, you can help ensure your kidneys stay healthy and function effectively.

If you have any further questions or concerns about kidney stones or health, don't hesitate to consult a healthcare professional. They can provide personalized advice and treatment plans tailored to your specific needs.

Stay hydrated, eat well, and keep learning about how to maintain your health. Here's to a future with healthy kidneys and a better understanding of kidney stones.

# Your feedback is greatly appreciated!

It's through your feedback, support and reviews that I'm able to create the best books possible and serve more people.

I would be extremely grateful if you could take just 60 seconds to kindly leave an honest review of the book on Amazon. Please share your feedback and thoughts for others to see.

To do so, simply find the book on Amazon's website (or wherever you purchased the book from) and locate the section to leave a review. Select a star rating and write a couple of sentences.

That's it! Thank you so much for your support.

**Review this product**

Share your thoughts with other customers

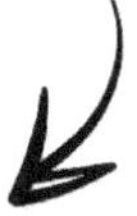

Write a customer review

# 22

# References

**Choices Senior Life.** (n.d.). *How to keep your kidneys healthy?* Retrieved from https://www.choiceseniorlife.com/how-to-kee p-your-kidneys-healthy/

**Comprehensive Urology.** (n.d.). *How to pass a kidney stone in 24 hours.* Retrieved from https://comprehensive-urology.com/uro logist-desk/how-to-pass-a-kidney-stone/

**Dr. Jeremy Kaslow, MD.** (n.d.). *Gout recommendations.* Retrieved from https://www.drkaslow.com/gout-recommendations

**Dreminozbek.** (n.d.). *Extracorporeal shock wave lithotripsy (ESWL) for urinary system stone disease.* Retrieved from https://d reminozbek.com/en/extracorporeal-shock-wave-lithottrypsy-eswl-for-urinary-system-stone-disease/

**Grace Laboratory.** (n.d.). *What is calculus in kidney?* Retrieved from https://gracelaboratory.com/what-is-calculus-in-kidney /

**Let's Get Checked.** (n.d.). *Protein intake and kidney damage: Can too much protein damage kidneys?* Retrieved from https://www.letsgetchecked.com/articles/can-too-much-protein-damage-your-kidneys/

**Lower Hunter Medical.** (n.d.). *Kidney stones: Management and dietary tips.* Retrieved from https://lowerhuntermedical.com.au/kidney-stones-management-and-dietary-tips/

**Mayo Clinic.** (n.d.). *Kidney stones – Symptoms and causes.* Retrieved from https://www.mayoclinic.org/diseases-conditions/kidney-stones/symptoms-causes/syc-20355755

**ModernTechBiz.** (n.d.). *What do kidney stones look like?* Retrieved from https://moderntechbiz.com/kidney-stones/what-do-kidney-stones-look-like/

**Muir Diablo Occupational Medicine.** (n.d.). *What to know about kidney stones and gallstones.* Retrieved from https://mdoccmed.com/articles/what-know-about-kidney-stones-and-gallstones

**National Kidney Foundation.** (n.d.). Retrieved from https://www.kidney.org/

**Neutech Medical.** (n.d.). *Renal ultrasound archives.* Retrieved from https://www.neutechmedical.com/tag/renal-ultrasound/

**Shyft Healthwatch.** (n.d.). *Listen to your body: Recognizing the signs of hyperuricemia.* Retrieved from https://www.betheshyft.com/healthwatch/listen-to-your-body-recognizing-the-sign

s-of-hyperuricemia/

**St. Luke's Health.** (n.d.). *Kidney stones causes and treatment.* Retrieved from https://www.stlukeshealth.org/services-special ties/urology/conditions/kidney-stones

**UPMC in Ireland.** (n.d.). *Kidney stones.* Retrieved from https://u pmc.ie/services/urology/conditions/kidney-stones

**Urology Care Foundation.** (n.d.). *What are kidney stones?* Retrieved from https://www.urologyhealth.org/urology-a-z/k/ kidney-stones

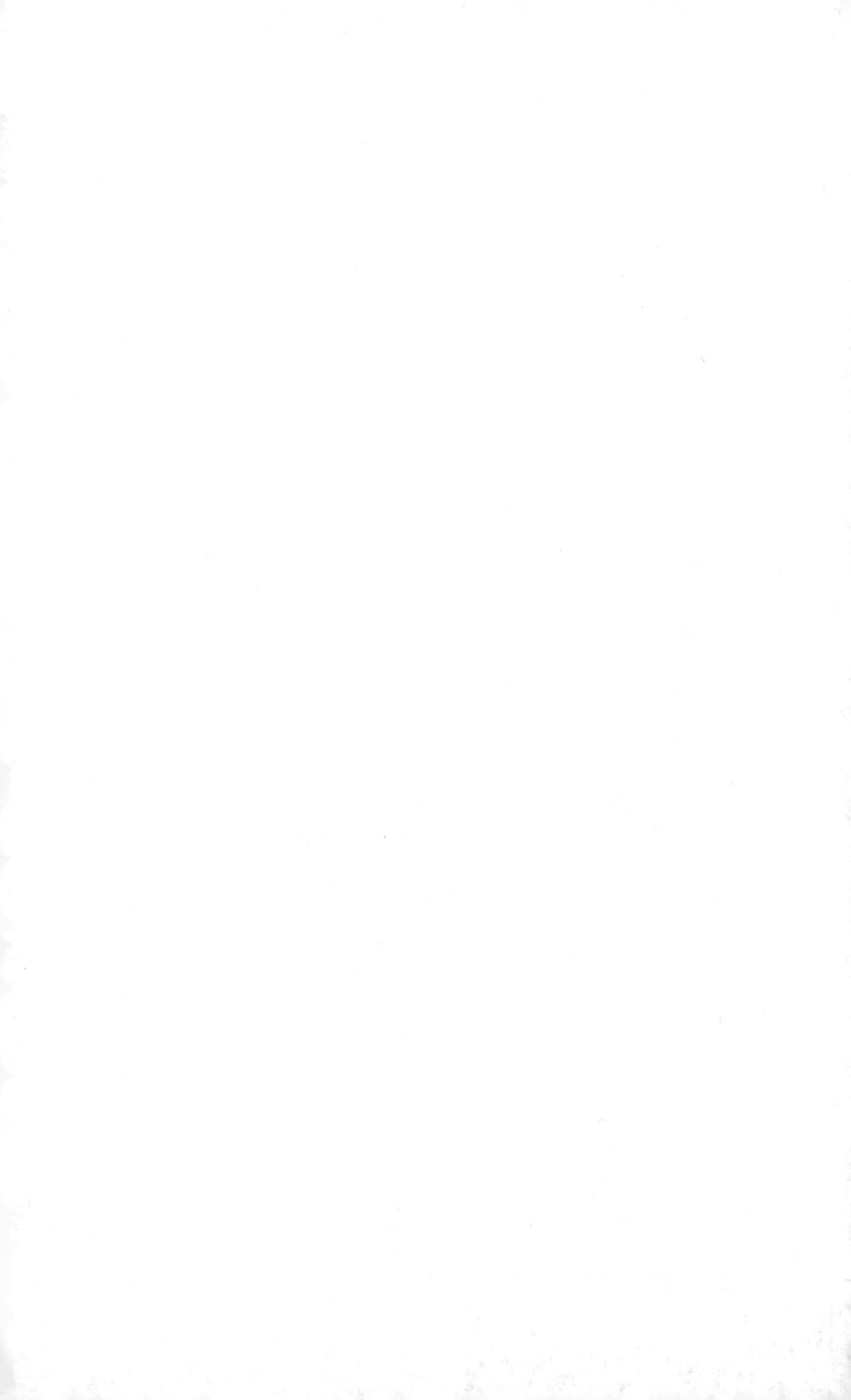